# Jailhouse Strong:

■  ■  ■

*The Successful Mindset Manual*

*Josh Bryant and Adam benShea*

Jailhouse Strong:
The Successful Mindset Manual

JoshStrength, LLC and Adam benShea
Copyright © 2014

ISBN-13: 9781502578990

# Introduction

The book, *Jailhouse Strong,* concludes with the Five Decrees:
1. Get Excited about Training
2. Get Plenty of Rest
3. Eat Meals at Regular Intervals
4. Stick to the Training Basics
5. When Conflict is Unavoidable, Strike First

When one journey ends, another may begin. While these decrees may be summarized as psychological mindset, recovery, nutrition, training methods, and self-defense, a deeper understanding of these principles will harden your body and sharpen your mind. In *Jailhouse Strong,* we offered a significant amount of information, and a number of examples, to demonstrate these decrees.

However, we realize that not all decrees are created equal. In particular, the right mindset is the fundamental element to becoming Jailhouse Strong. Without the necessary mental intention, physical training achievements (and self-preservation in adverse situations) will be difficult, if not impossible. This manual is about developing the successful mindset.

The successful mindset is one that takes you to your goals and out of physical, emotional, and mental imprisonment.

The successful mindset outlined in this manual will get your head straight and your mind right, so you can get bigger, better, and stronger.

When talking to people who trained behind bars, we found that physical training was the high point of a low point in their lives. In the institutional reality of life in an iron cage, many find a way to control their physical destiny by transforming their body into a hardened physique. Physical training can improve even the direst situation.

An incarcerated life can be characterized by long periods of mind-numbing monotony that are interrupted by momentary anxiety-inducing experiences.

Moreover, an incarcerated life may extend outside of the correctional facility. Imprisonment may take many forms, be it physical, mental, or spiritual. One can be imprisoned by the drab existence inside a cubicle farm as easily as they can be chained to a sedentary life focused on following social media updates. All such circumstances are categorized by their dull reality and a slow process toward inhibition of life.

In such conditions, many people look to speed up their lives. The office worker constantly checks the time, waiting to escape the confines of his job to the "freedom" of the local happy hour. The family man with the pressure of wife, kids, and in-laws yearns to watch SportsCenter in his man cave.

With this mindset, people are focused on killing time. However, as former con Daniel Genis noticed, "To kill your days is essentially to shorten your own life." Behind bars, time may become a nemesis or a resource. Those who become Jailhouse Strong use time as a resource to move toward the attainment of goals, physical and otherwise.

With this mindset, self-improvement becomes the focus of the day. Adherence to a rigorous physical training program is the most overt example of personal improvement. It offers a break from the redundant routine, and it promotes a level of emotional stability in an emotionally unstable environment.

Training becomes such a prized portion of a prisoner's day that many will avoid trouble so their yard workout privileges will not be revoked. Needless to say, nothing gets in the way of their workouts. This is the type of consistency that is the key for making any sort of serious gains.

With time, consistency, and discipline, you get stronger, mentally and physically. To become Jailhouse Strong, you set goals and you achieve them.

While prison guards are an easy example of a gate-keeper, there are "gatekeepers" on both sides of prison walls who will look to impede your progress toward goal achievement. You could have an incompetent, micromanaging boss who is threatened by your spreadsheet competency or a self-absorbed spouse who is jealous of your score in *Angry Birds.* In either case, the idea remains consistent: there will always be people who attempt to block your path toward success.

The acquirement of physical strength is the most readily available, and explicitly evident, means to combat the activities of the gatekeepers. Many cons have had limited, if any, success in life. With physical training, for the first time in their life they are able to command their own physical destiny. They are able to show anybody who sees them that they are able to use the tools of consistency and discipline to fill their time with productive activities; they achieve a sense of accomplishment.

A broad back and lean waist is a sign of success. This is not, however, a type of success that has to been limited to physical achievement. Rather, this physical success may be a metaphor—and a launching point—for success in any form.

No matter how great your physical strength may be, it will be useless if you are unaware of your potential for mental strength. When you are mentally and physically sharp, you've dramatically increased your chances of setting personal records and reigning victorious on the field, in the cage, in the alley behind the peeler bar, and in life. Becoming Jailhouse Strong has as much to do with mental strength as physical strength. To acquire real power, you must believe that you are powerful.

Let's talk about how you can do that.

## Growth versus Fixed Mindset

In her book, *Mindset: The New Psychology of Success,* Stanford psychologist Carol Dweck discusses the concepts of the fixed and growth mindsets.

People with the fixed mindset believe they are born winners or losers. They think that talent and intelligence are fixed traits. These individuals believe success is achieved via talent alone and not through hard work and development.

People with the fixed mindset like to revel in their greatness, instead of developing their talent. They ultimately fall short of their life's destiny because they worry about being embarrassed instead of focusing on becoming better.

The fixed mindset will never reach beyond its grasp.

In the growth mindset, people believe they are not born winners or losers, but choosers!

Perhaps the Western writer and rugged individualist, Louis L'Amour, explains this mindset best: "Up to a point a person's life is shaped by environment, heredity, and changes in the world about them. Then there comes a time when it lies within their grasp to shape the clay of their life into the sort of thing they wish it to be. Only the weak blame parents, their race, their times, lack of good fortune or the quirks of fate. Everyone has the power to say, 'This I am today. That I shall be tomorrow.'"

Through dedication and work ethic, anyone can develop both talent and intelligence to their limitless potential. The growth mindset spawns overachieving greatness.

In athletic performance, science demonstrates that when an athlete believes in his or her competition plan, the athlete is more likely to achieve success. The growth mindset aims at achieving any goal through a willingness to learn.

## A Desire to Learn

Everyone is born with an intense desire to learn. When placed in a new environment, a toddler will use all five senses to learn every little nuance about theirsurroundings.

People who embrace the will to learn experience success. As the world-renowned strength coach, Charles Poliquin, reminds us, "Learn more; earn more." Through learning you can attain spiritual, athletic, familial, or any other type of riches.

Learning, however, is a lifelong process. All too often, CEOs, for example, start off in the growth mindset as they work their way up the corporate ladder through mid-level and upper-level management positions with an intense desire to learn. They read the books, attend the seminars, and do everything in their power to learn as much as possible to fill their role as effectively as possible. They grow and the climb continues.

Somewhere along the way, many CEOs realize they have "arrived." No longer are they learners; they want to just look flawless. Looking smart and talented becomes the new objective. In turn, instead of hiring the best people for managerial positions, these CEOs feel threatened by subordinates looking smarter than them or getting credit for their own ideas.

Lee Iacocca nearly brought down Chrysler with this mindset; Kenneth Lay destroyed Enron with a similar outlook.

There is no such thing as resting on one's laurels; we are all moving forward or backward. We are always progressing or regressing; stagnation is a myth.

Without the growth mindset, the principles laid out in this book are impossible to implement.

## Developing a Growth Mindset

So what does it take to develop the growth mindset?

Embrace belief!

You must realize that your ultimate capabilities are morphological by way of hard and smart work and acquiring new pieces of knowledge and skills.

Embrace challenges!

The fixed mindset group hates challenges; it is scared of failure and believes failure indicates a lack of talent.

The growth mindset realizes that you can learn from challenges and they aid in personal growth. Challenges teach us and are paramount in the development of our arsenal of success.

Embrace hard work!

The fixed mindset views hard work and effort as a willful admission to a lack of talent.

Virtually every great athlete, musician, and businessman studies and practices his craft endlessly. Hard work and all-out effort is a given in the growth mindset. As Vince Lombardi said, "The harder you work, the harder it is to surrender."

View failure as learning!

The fixed mindset views failure as a lack of talent, or as an indication of lacking value at the core of self.

The growth mindset realizes failure is an opportunity to learn.

Thomas Edison said it best, "Every wrong attempt discarded is another step forward."

It is just as important to learn how not to do something as it is to learn how to do it. Do not be scared of failure. Embrace the Texas attitude toward failure. Instead of crying about the Alamo, Texans use "Remember the Alamo!" as their rally call. Painful defeats can catalyze victory.

There is no such thing as failure; there are only results!

Do not shy from criticism!

When it comes to criticism, the fixed mindset has a hard time admitting mistakes. Criticism, even in a constructive format, is seen as the ultimate form of an insult.

The growth mindset realizes that, although some criticism is mean-spirited and ill-conceived, it still offers a chance for growth. The growth mindset is open to feedback and suggestions.

Be inspired by success!

The fixed mindset views the success of others as a threat.

The growth mindset certainly does not shy away from competitiveness but realizes the success of others is a chance to receive inspiration and, more important, learn. People with this mindset find inspiration and learn from others who are successfully doing now what they want to do in the future.

People with the fixed mindset are chronic underachievers.

People with the growth mindset ultimately view themselves as "works in progress" and realize that their potential is developed over time.

Those with the fixed mindset do not play well with others, believing everyone is always out to get them.

By having the growth mindset, you realize that progress is experienced through active cooperation and learning from others.

Those with the fixed mindset destroy heroes. With cynicism and criticism, the fixed mindset will turn heroism into a tragedy.

Tabloids sell because people with this mindset want to see their favorite celebrities at their lowest point, at their most tragic. Rather than working to improve their own physical or emotional reality, the fixed mindset finds glimpses of cellulite and drinking binges comforting to their own stunted existence that falls fathoms short of the greatness waiting for them.

The growth mindset has a strong belief in heroes. By drawing inspiration from heroes, legends, and seemingly miraculous achievement, the growth mindset realizes there are still some things worth fighting for.

In whichever form of incarceration you find yourself, embrace the belief that you can grow, learn, and discover success.

# A Mindset of Success

## Motivation and Discipline for Mind Conditioning

Your goal is your portal to freedom from incarceration and you can achieve any goal you set for yourself. It just takes motivation. Motivation is the state of mind that generates positive feelings about achieving a purpose.

It also takes discipline. Discipline is what keeps you methodical in your actions as you strive to achieve your goal.

Your emotional state strongly dictates performance. Extreme depression, over-arousal, or fear can inhibit maximal performance. A focus on discipline is necessary for maximum performance.

The simplest way to bring focus and discipline to any endeavor is to follow those activities that put you in a state of bliss. The famous mythologist, Joseph Campbell, said that you should "follow your bliss and don't be afraid, and doors will open where you didn't know they were going to be." By following your bliss, you can find the path waiting for you and find the escape door leading out of your personal form of imprisonment.

Attack the pig iron or bang the heavy bag because it brings you bliss. Moreover, find your bliss and discipline will follow.

## The Pain-Pleasure Paradigm

Sometimes, however, an adherence to discipline requires that there will be times when you stray from immediate comforts. Following your bliss should not be confused with pursuing a life of permanent pleasure. According to Tony Robbins, pain and pleasure are the guides you use to make decisions on a daily basis. These can also serve as a guide for your goals in athletic performance, physical strength, or body composition.

For example, when you are dieting, what do you envision? What do you think about? Some view their diets as complete self-deprivation and torture. This is all they think about. Dieting is associated with pain and suffering. In the paradigm of pain and pleasure, these people view their diets within the spectrum of pain. Unless you are some sort of masochist, this is a quick path to failure. If the path to your goals is seen in a painful light, then more often than not, you will utterly fail.

In contrast, the people who succeed in dieting envision all the benefits that will come from their diet. For a bodybuilder it might be walking up to get the first-place trophy at a contest, for a college student it may be having the best body at spring break in Panama City, and for a fat guy it might just be envisioning himself talking to pretty girls with more confidence. These things all operate within the pleasure portion of this paradigm. All these are examples of people who choose to focus on the positive results of their desired outcomes, instead of the painful part of the process of getting there.

Here is a simple step-by-step method that uses discipline and inspires motivation to help you get what you want:

1. ***Define your goal clearly and write it down.*** *This means being specific about what you want. If you desire a better fight performance, what kind of improve-*

ments are you looking for? Do you want to increase your punching power and speed, or your grappling skills? Concentrate specifically on the actual aspect you wish to improve. Then write your goal down. You'll be surprised at how much clearer you can make it by simply putting it in words. When you have to select the exact words to define what you want, you develop a very clear image of your goal.

2. **Devise a series of short-term goals that will ultimately lead to realizing your main, or long-term, goal.** It's easier to attain a short-term goal that's within reach than to try and make great leaps and bounds of progress all at once. When you try too much at once and fail, you tend to get discouraged. Instead, set a number of short-term goals that you can accomplish and then knock them off one at a time. Focus exclusively on the goal you wish to achieve, not even thinking about the next short-term goal or the long run. With the completion of each one of your short-term goals, you will be closer to your major goal. And as you achieve your short-term goals, you motivate yourself to continue training.

3. **Create strategies for your success.** This is your game plan. On the same sheet that you wrote your long-term goal and listed the short-term goals that will get you there, you should break down your daily activities into the best means to get you where you're going. This means the routines, exercises, sets, reps, intensity, practice, rest periods, diet, and so on. Follow your own plan to success. Prepare a daily schedule that takes you in the direction you want to go. Keep your goal sheet current, and review it day by day.

4. ***Visualize yourself succeeding.*** *No one would attempt to build a house without a set of blueprints. Likewise, you must plan your success strategy and actually "see" yourself, in your mind's eye, accomplishing your goals. Your inner feelings, your thoughts, and your day dreams must all be filled with images of your ultimate success. Twice a day—once after training and once before bedtime—read your goal sheet out loud. Then close your eyes and with crystal clarity, see yourself performing perfectly, exactly as you want to. But see yourself actually accomplishing your goals, not just wistfully thinking about accomplishing them.*

5. ***Align your mind, body, and spirit with achievement.*** *By affirming your commitment to your stated goals and actually visualizing and verbalizing your commitment, you will find that your mind, body, and emotional self all become one (the YMCA was on to something powerful when it proclaimed "sound mind, body and spirit"). All three must be exercised in concert to produce synergistic results. The power of this union will send an emotional supercharge to your body by actually stimulating secretion of your body's emotion-producing endorphins. The alignment is accomplished by actually verbalizing your commitment while visualizing it. The central nervous system cannot tell the difference between a real and imagined experience. The more vivid and real your visualizations, the more the mind can work and the physiological mechanisms will follow. Repeat your commitment statement before, during, and after your success visualization every day.*

6. *Give yourself a reward for your accomplishments.*
*After you've achieved a short- or long-term goal, give*
*yourself a reward or treat of some sort. Buy yourself*
*new clothes or a needed item, or even a luxury one!*
*Reaffirm the good feeling in your mind and dwell upon*
*your achievement and your success. Congratulate*
*yourself and savor the feelings of pride and confi-*
*dence in having taken direct action to make yourself*
*better and stronger.*

## When Negative Addictions Become Positive Habits

The key to mental conditioning is to make your new thoughts and new approach a habit. The more regular your new habit becomes, the more quickly old and destructive habits fade away. Negative habits, or addictions (think smoking crack rock or playing excessive video games of sorcery and magic), may be replaced by a healthy habit (think throwing heavy weight around or grappling drills).

The only way to continue making progress is to regularly reinforce your new, goal-directed training. Remember the old adage, "Once is an accident; twice is a pattern."

It usually takes at least three weeks to implement this revised way of thinking and for your actions to become habits. During that time, you're likely to feel tempted to return to old patterns and habits. Don't do it! Focus on breaking through the incarceration of bad habits, rather than resigning yourself to a life imprisoned by these behaviors.

The more you resist old habits, the stronger you'll become, until you develop an iron will to succeed and you no longer even think about returning to those old habits.

Remember to create a goal, visualize it as real, and work regularly to attain it. You will get there!

To be the best fighter, weightlifter, or elementary school teacher, you need to see yourself in that light. This is not a feel-good exercise in futility. This will make your body produce literally drug-like effects that will help propel you to that next level.

Set a specific goal and strive for it! Man has a built-in success mechanism and does not operate efficiently without striving for a goal. Remember specificity—making more money is not a clear goal; making over six figures in a year is.

Once you establish your specific goal, you will need to stay motivated.

## Nine Steps to Getting and Staying Motivated

1. *Set short-term goals.*
2. *Let short-term goals lead you to the attainment of a long-term goal. Allow for occasional setbacks along the way, but regard them as learning experiences, thereby turning those setbacks into something positive.*
3. *Set a training schedule and stick to it. (A good place to find such a training program is in Jailhouse Strong.)*
4. *Make pain and fatigue work for you. Use them as signs that your all-out effort is helping you attain your goals.*
5. *Challenge yourself in your training.*
6. *Devise your own personal definition of success. It's what you say it is, not what someone else says it is.*
7. *Believe in yourself and foster positive aggression in your training.*
8. *Listen to your coach's advice and apply it to your workouts.*
9. *Build a strong ego, but a positively directed one.*

## The Incentive Factor

Motivation begins and ends with incentive—you have to know what you want and why you want it.

In *Jailhouse Strong*, this means focusing on the training habits that will free you from accepting the harsh imprisonment forced on you by a sometimes bitter reality. It could be iron bars, a nagging spouse, or a hectic work schedule.

In conditioning, this means you must train toward a specific improvement. More strength, speed, power, skill, endurance, or sheer muscle mass are various incentives, and they are part of larger incentives such as being liked and admired, being a winner or achiever, enjoying success, shaping a personal identity, gaining peer acceptance, and so on.

**2**

# The Powerful Mind

## Conditioning your Mind for Success

The mind and body are a team, and if you want to be a championship fighter or a top producing real estate broker you can never forget that. If you consistently visualize success, you will consistently succeed. To become a winner, you should practice the skill of "thinking like a winner."

We believe that anyone who has achieved great success in one area of their life can very easily achieve success in another area. Why? The expectations of success! After you becomes accustomed to acquiring success, you'll settle for nothing less. As a consequence, you will find that success begets success.

## Art Briles' Success Story

In 1988, Art Briles took over as the head football coach at Stephenville High School in Stephenville, Texas. Stephenville had not made the playoffs since 1952. By 1998, Briles had built Stephenville into a perennial powerhouse, making the playoffs every year since 1990, winning four state championships along the way, and setting multiple records in team offense. As a consequence, colleges took notice of Briles' success.

By being in the right place at the right time (something that seems to always happens to those who expect success), Briles took the job as running back coach at Texas Tech under the legendary Mike Leech and helped to revolutionize Tech's running game.

In the early 2000s, the University of Houston had developed a habit of losing, including a 0-11 season in 2001. Briles was offered the head coaching job. He embraced the opportunity and expected success. In his first year at the helm, U of H had a winning season, going 7-5.

By 2007, U of H had gone to three bowls in a row! In fewer than five years, Briles had taken arguably the worst Division I program in America to bowl games!

With Briles, one sees a pattern of success breeding success, and this pattern continued after his time at U of H. In 2007, Baylor offered Briles the job of taking over its failing football program, and it should not be a surprise that Baylor was in contention for a national championship in 2013.

Art Briles is a winner who expects success, and he makes a point to surround himself with "championship people." The success Briles has had at every level all started with an expectation of success. Having the right staff and the right recruits both helped over the long term, but none of this was in place his first year as head coach. Briles worked on himself first, and from there new success was inevitable.

From Briles, we can learn that when we expect success and have a dogged commitment to excellence, we find a way to be in the right place at the right time.

## Mental Preparation

Beyond physical conditioning, there is another kind of preparation that is just as important for achieving success. It's

9

one that involves subtle factors concerning your attitude and approach to competition.

Your ability to act and react spontaneously, with maximum power and proficiency, to any given situation in any discipline, is a major key to your conditioning and peak performance efforts.

You have to train and develop your attitude in order to develop the ability to "turn on" instantly and be able to do so with exceedingly great force. If you already have a positive mental outlook, then you have an excellent starting point for building and strengthening your mental capabilities.

You can achieve great things with your mind. The power of your mind can advance your physical training further and faster. It can also make the difference between winning and losing in competition, or in any aspect of life.

Mind power and successful mental conditioning come only with a sustained and sincere effort. You can't make a wish and hope it will come true and then forget about working on it. The mind reacts much the same way the body does. If you train and condition it regularly, it will respond with a performance you can always count on and be proud of.

Some of the key ingredients to an effective mind-conditioning program are motivation, incentive, visualization, and—most important of all—belief.

Studies show that when athletes believe in their competition training plans, they are more likely to be victorious in their given sport.

Just as winning is largely a mental process, a mental attitude, so is losing. Or, as Vince Lombardi once said, "Winning is not a sometime thing: it's an all the time thing. You don't win once in a while; you don't do things right once in a while; you do them right all the time. Winning is a habit. Unfortunately, so is losing."

You've no doubt heard of athletes being branded "losers." You've seen players "choke" when it comes down to the one crucial moment that will either make or break them. The ones who are broken are those who have failed to carry their training that extra step into the mental preparation necessary for victory.

What does this mean to you? It means *you've got to believe.*

You've got to believe in yourself, in your talents and capabilities, in your goals and all you hope to achieve and in your methods for achieving them. Believing and expecting success before you have achieved it is not make-believe. It is catalyzing a real physiological response. Expectations and beliefs augment the placebo effect; expecting success makes you a success-finding machine. A belief and expectation of success literally causes your brain to release chemicals that will act like drugs, but with the only side effect being success.

What if you took an attitude of success and expectancy toward achieving your goals? Even if you think this is unrealistic, do you think a pessimistic world view that attracts failure is more realistic? You have a choice about which attitude to take. Why not err on the side of expecting success?

The beginning of understanding what your mind holds in store for you is a simple realization. You must realize that within you is all the power you need to succeed—in training, competition, and life. Within you is all the potential for success. Within you is the brain power of a superman or superwoman.

As we said in *Jailhouse Strong,* "If there is one thing that you can take away from this book, it is this: you are born with everything you need to become Jailhouse Strong."

Once you make this realization—that you hold a vast wealth of knowledge, information, control, power, ability, and

11

potential—you can start to tap into that power. You can delve into your own secret depths and find out what you're really made of.

## Believe to Achieve: Is Placebo Your Drug of Choice?

"It might be a placebo effect but it's still an effect." —Chuck Liddell

The placebo effect is not akin to a belief in the make-believe; it is a real physiological response. The effect can be amplified according to the invasiveness of the placebo via the condition being treated, environment and the expectation of the participant receiving the placebo.

According to *The Journal of Medical Ethics,* placebo pain relief is a product of the release of endogenous opioids and endocannabinoids. In other words, your belief gives you a dose of morphine.

Expectations and beliefs augment the placebo effect: Expecting pain relief produces pain relief. A placebo literally causes your brain to release chemicals that will act like feel good drugs, without the chance of addiction or negative side effects. Belief can work like powerful drugs!

If you took this attitude of expectancy to being a great elementary school teacher, an elite fighter, or massive power-lifter, you will be more successful. Believe to achieve!

## Set Goals: Psychology is Physiology

"Psychology trumps physiology every time." —Alwyn Cosgrove

Psychology will directly influence physiology and how you perform.

Belief will boost your probability of success in any endeavor.

The *New England Journal of Medicine* published a study that examined the effectiveness of arthroscopic surgery on folks with arthritic knees. This study looked at 180 patients who received either arthroscopic surgery on their knee or a placebo surgery. In other words, while some of these patients received legitimate surgery, others received an inconsequential skin incision that tricked them into believing surgery was performed.

Subsequently, patients were examined for improved levels of pain and improved function over a 24-month period. Both the surgery group and the placebo group improved postop and "post imagined op." At no point did the surgery group report less pain or better function than the placebo group! Both believed and both achieved.

This study has implications far beyond examining the efficacy of arthroscopic surgery. If you believe, you achieve.

If the right mindset can produce the same results as surgery, it's time to put your beliefs under the knife and transform yourself into the purpose-driven, goal-striving being you were created to be.

**3**

*Competition*

## Pre-Contest Anxiety

After all of the grueling training and conditioning, the time comes down to competition day, be it golf, cage fighting, or an interview for your dream job.

Remember, you do not need to put on pads, gloves, or a helmet to be competitive. Competition emerges when there is something that matters. You prepare for competition by sacrificing and working toward the goal that will bring the freedom of success.

You have dedicated yourself to becoming the best you can be, and, in the process, you may have completely destroyed any social life you once had. Yes, all this dedication and sacrifice has been for this single day of reckoning!

While many have worked hard and prepared themselves more than adequately physically, they fail to live up to their potential.

Why? They aren't prepared mentally.

Everyone experiences at least some level of anxiety, or what's often known as "jitters," before a bout. It's only natural. Not only that, but a small case of nerves can sometimes be a plus to your performance, as it summons up a fresh supply of adrenaline and gives you a little extra boost to face the competition. It's called being "psyched."

But nerves, anxiety, and jitters can be destructive, too.

In fact, if you're not prepared mentally, you can think yourself right into defeat. In this way, you could reach a state of "analysis paralysis."

It isn't easy to control your mind's response to pressure. Everyone reacts differently. Some thrive on pressure situations and always come through; others shake and lose control and falter.

While few of us are completely free of tension, there are some commonsense approaches that can effectively reduce tension in your life.

## The Pre-Start Phenomenon

Many psychological factors converge at the time of a major competition. Pressure mounts. The athlete wants to succeed, to do well, to triumph. Yet there is also that creeping doubt, that fear of failure, that worry that everything will go wrong or that the competition will prove to be overwhelming.

If that happens to you, what can you do about it?

First, pinpoint the source of your anxiety.

You could be afraid of many things. Is your girlfriend watching you perform? Are you worried about letting down your coach? There is also the fear of pain due to possible injury, the fear of a group turning against you for your poor performance, and a host of other factors.

These kinds of fears produce instant physical reactions. Your heart rate increases, adrenaline flows, you may feel muscularly tense, and if the fear lasts awhile, it could keep you from sleeping.

It's natural to have anxiety, but if you allow an excess of it to control your mind and thoughts, then it may be more deeply rooted than the simple fear of failure. So dig down and unearth this fear.

Second, identify the worst case scenario.

Fear works from a foundation of uncertainty and under a shroud of mystery. It is easier to fear that which you do not know or understand. Once the foundation of fear is unearthed and the shroud lifted, the power of fear to control your imagination is reduced greatly.

Identifying your worst case scenario allows you to come to terms with that which can lead to your demise. Like the samurai who meditated daily on the prospect of their death, you can reach a level of emotional equilibrium when you come to terms with the possibility of this scenario.

Last, be willing to achieve success.

Lots of people have a fear of failure. But some athletes also have the fear of success! Success can include a heavy load. You may wonder if people will now expect more from you and if you can live up to their new expectations. With success, there tends to be the expectation of better results. You should not worry about that; you should focus on what you expect from yourself.

The comedian Bill Cosby may have said it best: "I don't know the key to success, but the key to failure is trying to please everybody." Concerning yourself with other people's expectations leads to failure; again, focus on what you expect from yourself and implement a plan to get there.

With all of your fears and concerns, it is possible that you simply have the game or event too much on your mind. In this state, called the pre-state phenomenon, you are too aroused, and this can cause stress. To combat this pre-start phenomenon, you must practice what are known as stress reduction techniques, or more specifically, arousal control techniques.

## Arousal Control Techniques

Stress should never be allowed to get the better of you. A little stress is okay, but a lot of it can cause physical dysfunction. Remember that stress begins and ends in the mind. You must strive to mobilize your mental forces at the appropriate point, which is usually just before the competition begins. Here are some tips for controlling tension:

1. **Be careful not to peak too soon.** *Be well prepared, but save your best effort for the actual competitive outing and let out all your energy then, not before.*

2. **Be wary of too much activity during the pre-start period.** *Too much agitation and nervous energy release can work against you, sapping your reserves and creating greater mental anxiety.*

3. **Avoid emotional contagion from other athletes in the pre-start period.** *It's easy to be influenced by someone else's nervousness or anticipatory response. Don't let that happen. If necessary, remove yourself from the group, even if it's only a "mental closeout."*

4. **Be aware of your emotional state at the end of your contest,** *as this is often what you bring with you to preparation for your next competition. Instead of looking at the negative aspects, try to bring a positive feeling with you from your effort, your results, and your improvements. Bottom line: Every time you compete, you gain experience regardless of the outcome.*

## Psyching Up

"Psyching up" refers to what is done in the start period, immediately preceding the competitive outing. Remember, too much psyching up can be devastating to your performance.

You've heard of the athlete who's been "psyched out" by his opponent. That means his mind was affected, which led to his losing performance. But you can also psych yourself out by thinking too much about what might happen in the event itself.

Tremendous tension can build to the point of escalating fatigue when you psych yourself up too much. The simple remedy for this is to remove yourself from the warm-up and retire to a quiet area where you can practice some of the "mind control" techniques referred to earlier.

In addition, there is tremendous benefit in using humor to reduce the terror or anxiety caused by a looming fight.

As the Beat stage performer Lord Richard Buckley used to say, "Humor is the absence of terror, and terror the absence of humor." In this sense, terror refers to the mind's capacity to frighten itself. To combat the potential for self-induced mental panic, many athletes like to surround themselves with a training team that is able to keep the training hard, but the mood lighthearted. Therefore, it is not uncommon to enter the locker room of a top-level MMA fighter before a fight and find an environment that resembles an amateur comedy hour.

Now psyching up for competition is not unnatural or abnormal. In fact, it's necessary to some degree. All good athletes must mentally prepare themselves for a contest shortly before it's about to begin. About two to five minutes before your game or event, you should be practicing psyching methods, but in a controlled and calm manner.

The truly great athletes always seem to possess an outward calm, no matter how intense their inner psyching is at the moment. They have a single-minded focus on what they are about to do. They don't need to jump up and down and bash heads, slap faces, or growl like an animal. All their base and primordial instincts are gathering inside of them for a controlled source of raw power. They will let it all out only when the bell rings and the competition demands it.

## The Emotional State of the Competitor

Your mind and your emotions are tightly tied together. It's up to you, as the competitor, to find a balance between them and exert control over them.

Your emotional state plays a large role in your overall performance. The way you are feeling inside has repercussions for your behavior and performance on the outside.

Many different factors go into the makeup of a solid emotional base. Some of these factors are personal life, sex life, family life, job, daily schedule, diet, financial matters, health concerns, and most important, self-esteem.

Your own self-esteem contributes greatly to the level of your sports performance. Self-esteem can vary greatly within the time confines of a single athletic event, and it can mean the difference between winning and losing. One minute you may hate yourself over an error you've committed in the cage, and a few moments later you could reverse that feeling completely by throwing an exceptional kick to the head and knocking your opponent out! This can be referred to as momentum, but it's just as valid when you call it self-esteem. An athlete's mental appraisal of himself counts for a great deal in his performance.

## Fear and Self-Esteem

Fear, depression, and anxiety or over-arousal can all lead to a sub-par performance on any field of play. For every winner, there is a loser, and often the distinguishing feature between the two is attitude, positive thinking, and the absence of inhibiting fear.

Fear of the competition, for instance, can put you in a defeatist frame of mind even before the fight begins. If you're so "psyched out" that you consider your opponent unbeatable, then you have defeated yourself.

This is described best in the movie *Rocky V*, when Rocky is talking to a young pupil about fear: "You see, fear is a fighter's best friend... but the thing is, you gotta learn how to control it. 'Cause fear is like this fire and it's burning deep inside. Now, if you control it, Tommy, it's gonna make you hot. But, you see, if this thing here controls you, it's gonna burn you and everythin' else around you up."

Your goal is to foster belief in yourself, train hard to achieve the means to victory, and then realize you have made your belief work for you.

All of your successes begin with the belief in yourself. In fact, belief and success go hand in hand. Once you control your fear, you begin to see yourself as potentially better than your opponent, and that's the key to winning!

In an uncontrolled state of fear, you will never see yourself as potentially better than your opponent. So it's obvious then that your state of mind determines, to a large extent, whether or not you ever "see" victory.

Fear of injury is another inhibiting factor.

You have probably heard of the term "oft-injured," which refers to the athlete who is forever on the disabled list. Sometimes, when returning to active play, this athlete tends to be gun-shy, afraid of injury, and might even alter the style of play to prevent injury. Ironically, playing to protect yourself against injury often leads to it. This is because you're pulling up, contracting your muscles irregularly, and not following through with movements. You are focusing on the injury instead of the game. It is not by chance that the NFL players who play a decade straight without missing a game are also the hardest hitters (think 1970s Pittsburgh Steelers offensive lineman Mike Webster and his mentor, Ray Mansfield).

## Visualization: Mental Training in Strength Training

The world-renowned biomechanist Vladimir Zatsiorsky contends that most people use about 65 percent of their muscles' potential strength, but trained weightlifters can use 80 percent in training and potentially 90 percent in competition. The right mindset is critical to lifting heavy weight.

Under the threat of potential danger, the mind can push the body to attain inconceivable accomplishments. Austin Smith, a 15-year-old Michigan teen, lifted the front end of a 2,000-pound car off of his 74-year-old grandpa. A skinny kid, he was able to do this by "committing to the pull." Directed focus allowed him to pull an unbelievable deadlift.

You do not need to go into a life-or-death state of psychosis every training session, because too much fatigue could be imposed on your central nervous system. Training with a focused, aggressive attitude can get you to that 80 percent range of total strength. Continued focus may even get you into the 90 percent range during competition.

Max effort strength is the largest amount of force that can be produced under voluntary conditions. Absolute strength is the greatest force that can be produced under involuntary conditions, measured in a laboratory setting.

Approaching absolute strength is nearly impossible, something most people will never scratch the surface of. However, the right mindset can serve as your game changer! In Mel Siff's monumental classic *Supertraining,* he writes about how the development of strength is related to the number of muscle fibers firing simultaneously, which is entirely a function of the nervous system. Guided mental imagery, or self-talk, to produce more rapid efforts can recruit a great number of muscle fibers at a faster rate of firing. The result is lifting more weight.

Focus on the task at hand and visualize yourself succeeding. Take 20 minutes a day to relax and watch a mental movie of yourself and your future successes. Remember this is accomplished through breathing deeply and relaxing; the more vivid the movie, the more real the experience. Whether you're a stock market tycoon or an elite athlete, the more real the experience, the more transferable the level of success.

Brain activity precedes movement, and it is vital to visualize correct movements long before those movements are performed. Visualization techniques were utilized by top Russian and Eastern Bloc weightlifting coaches for decades before receiving more widespread acceptance in the Western world. No two great fighters fight exactly the same; no two deadlifters move a weight in exactly the same fashion. Being able to visualize your optimal technique is crucial to achieving that most coveted Soviet title, "master of sport."

## Concentration

Success in the cage can almost be likened to the practice of Zen masters. The concentration is so complete that there is no consciousness of concentration. The player must be one with his sport in order to execute it to optimal ability.

You may have been in a situation where your attention was so rapt and absorbed in one thought that you completely blocked out all others. This was probably due to your high concentration level on some thought of great importance to you. In the 1980s pop culture classic *Top Gun,* Charlie (played by Kelly McGillis) asks Maverick (played by Tom Cruise) what he was thinking while engaged in aerial combat. To which Maverick responds: "You don't have time to think up there. If you think, you're dead." Thinking, rather than acting, during an airborne dogfight has dire consequences. Similarly, to achieve success on the deadlift platform, or while navigating your way through the barbed wire portion of a mud race, you must have complete concentration.

You cannot be thinking of extraneous factors while putting forth maximal effort. The best performances are nearly always those that are executed just below total consciousness. After knocking out an opponent, boxers commonly report a lack of event consciousness. They had essentially retreated into their own inner mind, where there is no pain or discomfort and where only positive forces loom.

In the antiquated world of the samurai, this was called "mindfulness." When you are in a state of mindfulness, you are aware of all that surrounds you, but all that is around you does not deter the focus that is within you.

There is, in fact, a degree of luxury that comes with the opportunity to disregard, and be free from, cerebral concerns. The legendary Brazilian Jiu Jitsu fighter Rickson Gracie calls this a "zero point." It is a place where you rely on intuition to act and react. It can be understood as a type of existential bliss where you are open to live totally in the moment.

The opportunity to escape from the cluttered mental space where we spend the majority of our days can be addictive. It is for this reason that many become addicted to those activities that push cognitive processes beyond the normative functioning mode. You become hooked on living in, and for, that moment of complete concentration.

This kind of focus is not just addictive; it can also be a confidence builder. The more you focus on what you're working to achieve, the fewer distractions will enter your awareness. This lifts you out of the state of mind where you can't "see" success and puts you in a place to achieve success. Once you begin to see success, you consider yourself potentially better than the competition. Little by little, you concentrate more and more, until you're unaware of anything in your way. You see your clear path to victory and success.

This is total concentration. It is this kind of total concentration that comes to those who develop total self-confidence. You must have high self-esteem and high motivation, while remaining consistent in your training and sports-conditioning program.

You must develop your mind conditioning to the point that total concentration is merely a learned response, one you never consciously think about anymore.

In some sports, we have heard coaches assure their athletes that, no matter what happens, your opponent is not going to beat you up if you lose. In combat sports (from Sanshou Chinese Kickboxing to informal slap boxing matches), though, your opponent does beat you up if you lose. The potential for an ass kicking does provide a much higher degree of anxiety. As a consequence, the threat of physical violence may necessitate a deeper and sharper form of mental concentration. In fact, with an intentional mindset, one can use the risk of physical harm as a motivational aid for focusing on the direction toward success.

The ability to turn trial and tribulation into triumph is an essential component of the successful mind.

In much the same way that noncontact sports may provide some a degree of security, sports like basketball or football may provide a degree of comfort in knowing you have teammates to help you achieve victory. For the sake of survival, humans are pack animals; communal living offers security, safety, and support. MMA fighters, powerlifters, and dwarf tossers all have teams, training partners, sparring partners, and coaches (dwarf tossers even have a union), but their team cannot assist the athlete in the cage, on the platform, or in the smoke-filled corner of your local mobile home turned bar where the largely forgotten (and often illegal) sideshow act of little person throwing is practiced every other Thursday night to the glee of performer and audience alike.

On the one hand, without the comfort of a team behind you, the circumstances that are confronted by a solo individual may increase stress. On the other hand, without the need to concern oneself with the needs of others, the individual is allowed the luxury of concerning himself solely with his own performance.

Again, the ability to turn trial and tribulation into triumph is an essential component of the successful mind.

Once the cage locks, it is all you. Individual sports cause much higher degrees of anxiety. Couple that fact with large crowds and an opponent who wants to physically harm you, and it is easy to let your emotions get out of control.

Ever wonder why, in low-level professional boxing, it is not uncommon to see an old club fighter, who appears to be out of shape, defeat a young stud? The old club fighter makes a living off these young studs because after going through the motions of the fight so many times, he is able to control his anxiety, whereas the young and inexperienced ones haven't yet learned to master volatile emotions.

You can punch harder, kick harder, and take more punishment if you are in the right mental state. Specifically, how fast you can punch, shoot in, or kick is influenced by the number of motor units you can recruit collectively as quickly as possible. According to the biomechanist Mel Siff, this is closely related to *personal motivation* and biofeedback techniques. That is, guided mental imagery or self-talk may recruit a great number of muscle fibers at a faster rate of firing. This means harder, faster strikes, takedowns, and submissions.

We can't over emphasize the degree to which mental preparation is often overlooked in MMA, powerlifting, mud runs, and all sports for that matter.

In sports that require maximum skill, speed, endurance, and strength while adhering to stringent rules, mental preparation can prove invaluable. If you don't follow the referee's commands or you let rage take control and violate a rule, guess what happens? Possibly a disqualification, and that's counted as a loss on your record! Moreover, an enraged mind will cloud your ability to properly execute the intricacies of the techniques that illustrate your combat ability.

In regard to this, training is for mental and physical preparation, and the contest is where you get to demonstrate your hard work. Without proper transference between training and demonstration in the cage, a fighter will never be at his best.

Your conscious mind deals with things at face value, such as reasoning, logic, communications, and things of that nature. Most people believe they operate only in this part of their mind. But this part of your mind is only a small percentage of your total mental capacity.

The subconscious mind directly influences your concept of self, which directly affects your anxiety levels and how well you can fight. The power to achieve and do great things is in your subconscious mind. The simple truth is, once again, you must believe in order to achieve.

In the 1950s, clinical and experimental psychologists proved that the human nervous system is unable to differentiate between a real experience and a vividly imagined and detailed experience. This does not mean that you can repeat 10 times a day, "I will be a champion in the UFC," and it will happen. That would be a passive experience.

For the nervous system to believe it is doing what you are imagining, you must create a vivid mental movie complete with the feelings, sights, sounds, and smells that would accompany the experience in real life. You need active experiences to positively affect your subconscious mind.

The discovery of a sense of self can help in training. Additionally, it can aid your competitive performance.

In the January 1959 issue of *Cosmopolitan* magazine, T. F. James was quoted as saying, "Understanding the psychology of the self can mean the difference between success and failure, love and hate, bitterness and happiness."

According to Maxwell Maltz, our triumphs, failures, and other people's reactions to these triumphs and failures form our concept of self. In other words, our experiences shape our self-image. It isn't so much the actual experiences but the way we perceive these events.

The good news is that the human nervous system can't tell the difference between real and imagined experiences, which means that you can train mentally to defeat opponents in your subconscious mind that you may not yet have physically defeated.

Here's an example. Johnny is a local-level MMA a fighter with a .500 record. If Johnny believes he is just a mediocre local-level fighter, then he is precisely that. But if Johnny believes he is a rapidly progressing fighter on his way to a championship, the odds of his becoming good are greatly increased. Another good example of this is when a fighter, an athlete, or an aspiring runway model makes excuses and blames his genetics for his lack of performance. Genetics are one piece of the equation, but how many people have reached their genetic potential? In fact, few have even come close.

To be successful in any aspect of your life, you have to have a positive self-image. Most efforts to change one's self-image are directed at the superficial level with too-often-bogus self-esteem programs. In order to achieve positive gains, we must transform at the core of our being. Once we alter our self-image, it's easier to accomplish things within the realm of this new self-image.

Prescott Lesky, considered one of the founding fathers of self-image psychology, conceived personality as a system of ideas that seem to maintain consistency with one another. Thoughts and goals that are inconsistent with this system of ideas are not acted upon, while ideas aligned with this system are acted upon. Lesky emphasized that at the nucleus of this system of ideas is an individual's concept of self.

To borrow from Maltz, the creative mechanism within every individual is impersonal. It can work automatically to achieve success or failure. Yet this depends on the goals you set for yourself. Present it with positive goals and the "success mechanism" will set in. Present it with negative goals and the "failure mechanism" will set in. Our goals are mental images developed in the conscious mind. The key is a realistic, positive self-image.

From this view, every living thing has a goal-striving mechanism put there by God to sustain life. A bear born in the spring has never experienced winter, yet somehow knows in the fall to prepare for hibernation. People have these innate abilities not only for sustaining life, but also for achieving great things in life, if desired.

The great Scottish philosopher Dugold Stewart once said, "The faculty of imagination is the great spring of human activity and the principal source of human improvement." That old Scotsman was on to something.

The use of mental imagery doesn't just start before a competition. If you wish to be the best, imagery should become a regular component of training. Know what your current goal is and know, without a doubt, that you will accomplish it. After that, look to the future. Find a new target and plan on how you will achieve that next goal.

Maxwell Maltz reminds us that man is a goal-oriented being; he is engineered that way. This means you must set specific goals for your fights and training. Training goals need to be specific, measurable, and realistic. Goals need to be established for the micro, meso and macro training cycles. That is, you need to have a plan for the short, medium, and long term. Each phase has a unique goal that helps you achieve the ultimate goal of reigning victorious on the mat, in the boardroom, or wherever.

Want to win your next contest or surpass a personal best? Where do you want to be a year from now?

Answering "Yes" or "Doing my best" is not a proper goal. It isn't specific enough. Give your brain a detailed and specific target (goal) you want to achieve, and watch what happens!

Men are hardwired to achieve goals and conquer obstacles. As John Patrick Mason (played by Sean Connery) in the movie *The Rock* says: "Losers always whine about their best. Winners go home and screw the prom queen." Losers make excuses about their jobs, money, or training partners while the winners go out and find success.

Brain activity precedes movement, and it is vital that correct movements are visualized long before those movements are performed. In fact, along with mass-produced vodka and the Kalashnikov assault rifle, being able to visualize your optimal technique may have been the greatest development in the Spartan world of the old Soviet Eastern Bloc.

## The Mental Imagery Program

As mentioned earlier, each day, set aside 20 minutes for mental imagery training, or what you can think of as your "movie." Find a dark, comfortable place to lie down and relax your muscles. This should be a place where all the anxieties and troubles of everyday life can be forgotten.

Start developing a movie in your head, a movie where you are the star. Successful visualizations benefit from as many details as possible. Visualize yourself arriving at the event location, psyching up, and performing your warm-up drills with relative ease.

If you're an MMA fighter, see yourself walking to the cage, entering the cage, looking across the cage at your opponent, and then using your best techniques to neutralize and overcome him.

Finally, visualize yourself in the middle of the cage with your hand raised in victory. You should use all your senses to make the visualization as true to real life as possible. Hear the crowd, smell the concession stand, and feel the cage's canvas under your bare feet.

This experience should be like a vivid dream, the kind where you wake up and feel it has actually happened. You want your central nervous system to have a real experience. After experiencing this vivid dream, the real life experience may seem like déjà vu. You have already experienced this. Your subconscious mind says so, and that is where the power of achievement lies!

Many successful fighters actually practice the art of walking to the cage with a high degree of confidence. Additionally, they have simulated experiences of victory in the cage. Playing the physical part of their mental visualization, they progress through the pending fight and include an ending where the coach or trainer raises their hand in victory (just as they intend the referee to do in the near future).

In private conversation, powerlifting legend Garry Frank once said: "When I walk up to the platform, the lift has already been done in my mind. I'm just doing the required going through the motions." Visualization must be part of your daily routine throughout your entire training cycle. Training lifts have built the foundation, but unless performed under competitive circumstances, they are meaningless. Mental imagery is where an athlete bridges the gap. The goal should not be to equal training lifts. It should be to exceed them.

Visualize every detail of the meet—warming up, time between attempts, approaching the platform, and making your lifts "nine for nine." Visualize the people coming up to you after the meet and congratulating you.

Coauthor Josh Bryant had a particular visualization technique for achieving a new deadlift personal record. Two to three times a week he would load his goal weight for the upcoming meet. He put the weight on the bar, played his favorite music, and visualized himself lifting that weight. Sometimes he approached the weight and gave it a good shake, reminding himself that come meet day, gravity no longer held supremacy but Josh Bryant did. He set aside 15 minutes for this activity, but many times it lasted for a couple of hours. The first time he deadlifted 800 lbs. in a meet, he easily bested his previous best of 749. This was due to his mental preparation, which made the extra 51 lbs. a cinch.

Visualization is not accomplished through strain or effort. Instead, it's achieved through relaxation. Try to systematically relax your muscles, one muscle group at a time. Then start to develop the movie in your head. Play back in your mind your past successes, like a successful competition or any event that was positive.

Reflecting on past victories and successes is helpful in defining a positive self-image. The key is to help these positive experiences build a foundation for your psyche. Realize, with proper focus, that the future will look better, and you will begin to appreciate the past with a degree of healthy nostalgia.

Louie Pasteur once said, "Chance favors the prepared mind." Napoleon Bonaparte role-played, and so did General Patton. Both these men were ready for almost any situation that could arise because they had mentally prepared for these scenarios.

Envision yourself not only as a big time athlete but also as a "big deal." As you win more competitive outings, people will be coming to you for advice. Envision your new role as one of your chosen sports elite, and the admiration and notoriety that accompany this new status.

If you have the freedom, it can be helpful to decorate your workout facility. Posters of past greats can serve as a great motivational tool. You should have heroes you admire and who will motivate you to become better.

Today's training methods are far more advanced than those of yesteryear, so you can conceivably surpass those heroes. Just remember, they were way ahead of their time for their era. Be thankful they paved the way for you, and never lose respect for them.

Psychologists tell us that even the color of your training facility can have an effect on your psyche. Psychologists have linked red to aggressive behavior; this may be beneficial to some, but it may encourage the already aggressive types negatively. For them, calming blue is a better choice. Find what works for you. Former UFC welterweight champion Matt Hughes has his gym designed in camouflage, which gives a feeling of combat to his training.

You now know how to create a positive self-image, but what about negative people and the negative energy they bring? If you can distance yourself from these negative energies, that's your best bet. If you can't, simply pay them no mind.

Do not hate these people, because hate and contempt breed resentment, and resentment, in and of itself, is a negative energy. Remember, the opposite of hate is not love, but apathy. Let the negative people go on their journey and you keep going on yours. Let your energy flow in a positive direction, and not in the direction of someone you don't like. Save all the energy for yourself and the ones you love.

## Relaxation

In combat sports, it is not uncommon to hear trainers tell their trainees to just relax. But it's hard to relax when someone is attempting to take your head off! Relaxation doesn't mean taking a laid-back approach. In this context, it means eliminating unnecessary movements and eliminating the expenditure of unnecessary energy. In running, this is called "fuel economy."

A study by Schucker, Hagemann, Strauss and Volker (2009), titled "The Effect of Attentional Focus on Running Economy," showed that "overthinking" running movements has a negative effect on fuel economy. In relation to pugilism, ask yourself who you think will fatigue faster: a relaxed boxer who, when the time is right, automatically throws a right cross? Or the one who has to think about every movement associated with the punch?

A great way to reach this desired level of relaxation is to understand the importance of being happy in your chosen profession. When you look at the looming moment of competition as an opportunity to showcase your growing skill set, you will be happy and grateful for the occasion. With a growing fondness, you will look forward to the day when you have the chance to perform.

Remember the words of the former heavyweight boxing champion Mike Tyson: "There's nothing more deadly or more proficient than a happy fighter. Everybody believes the mean, and the surly fighter, is the tough fighter, but that's not true. The guy who's most relax[ed] and loves what he does, and is happy to be in there doing what he does."

When you have the opportunity to showcase your success, revel in the moment and broadcast your skillset.

# *Closing Thoughts*

Do not forget: You already have all you need to become Jailhouse Strong. That is, you carry the tools for physical and mental power. You have the skill set to find success.

The initial step is to find what you want and make a goal of achieving success. With motivation, discipline, and hard work you can break past any obstacles, gate keepers, and constraints standing in your way. Remember that the instances of falling short of your goals are temporary results that can feed future success.

Success takes many forms. It may be the outward manifestation of power presented by Jailhouse Strong bulk. It can be achieved in the more subtle intellectual, spiritual, and financial realms as well. In whichever realm you find your goals, work toward success, regardless of how high the walls surrounding your current reality.

51471090R00027

Made in the USA
Lexington, KY
25 April 2016